I0555227

Praise
Through The Pain

Diagnosis to Destiny

by

ANGEL FAULK
"The Fitness Angel"

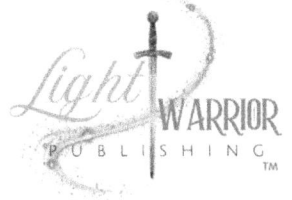

Praise Through the Pain: Diagnosis to Destiny ©2025 Angel Faulk

Light Warrior Publishing: Nashville, TN

Paperback ISBN: 978-1-969202-06-3

Hardback ISBN: 978-1-969202-08-7

Ebook ISBN: 978-1-969202-07-0

Editor: Elizabeth M. Charle with Polished Point Editing

Cover Design: Tammy Largin

All scriptures from the *New International Version* (NIV) *Holy Bible, New International Version*®, NIV® Copyright ©1973, 1978, 1984, 2011 by Biblica, Inc.® Used by permission. All rights reserved worldwide permission. All rights reserved worldwide.

Disclaimer: This book is for informational and educational purposes only and is not intended as medical advice. Always consult with your physician or other qualified health care provider before beginning any exercise program, dietary changes, or health plan. The author and publisher disclaim any liability for injury or adverse outcomes resulting from the use of the information contained herein.

To my husband, Wade—
a steadfast presence, a well of wisdom,
anchoring me through every season,
steady and sure when I dream beyond the horizon.

To my children, Lydia and Ethan, and my son-in-law, Josh—
whose courage and dreams
light my heart with hope and joy,
walking boldly in the purpose God has laid before you.

And to Jesus—
my Savior, my best friend, my rock, and my healer,
whose grace carries me through every trial and triumph,
whose unfailing love is the promise of new beginnings.

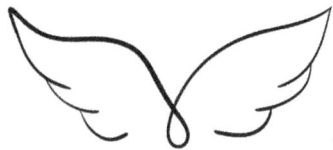

Table of Contents

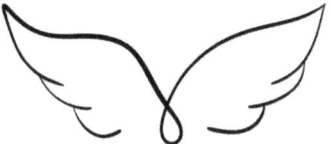

Introduction

*A*t fifty-six years old, I reflect on a journey that has been anything but ordinary. For nearly thirty years, I've taught fitness, empowering others to transform their lives. But my own transformation began with an unexpected and life-altering challenge—a brain tumor that nearly took everything from me, including my life. After surgery, I had to relearn how to walk, talk, and swallow. The tumor left me with facial paralysis, forcing me to confront something I never anticipated: a new identity as a woman.

For someone who had spent decades in the fitness industry, where appearance often feels tied to self-worth, this was and still is a deeply humbling experience. I had to remind myself that true beauty comes from within. It was during this time of recovery and soul-searching that I leaned on my faith more than ever. God reminded me of one of His promises: I am fearfully and wonderfully made (Psalm 139:14, NIV). Those words became my anchor as I rebuilt not only my face and body but also my spirit.

My recovery led me to learn about nutrition because I wanted to heal. To aid in the process, I embraced a plant-based lifestyle, joining a wellness company that taught me the incredible healing properties of plants. Although not comparable to a life-threatening brain tumor, life then threw another curveball, menopause. This pivotal moment shifted my perspective on nutrition, introducing me to the importance of protein and animal foods in building strength and vitality. Through trial and error, I found balance—a diet rich in protein while still celebrating the abundance of fruits and vegetables.

Today, I run a thriving coaching business dedicated to helping women rediscover their health, navigate menopause, lose fat, and build muscle through high-protein diets complemented by nutrient-rich plants. My mission is simple: to empower women to reclaim their health and strength during one of life's most transformative phases.

This book is not just about my story. It's about the faith-filled lessons learned along the way —the science behind fitness and nutrition, the mindset shifts required for change, and the strategies that can help you achieve your goals. Whether you're facing a serious diagnosis, going through menopause, or simply seeking better health, this journey is proof that no obstacle is insurmountable.

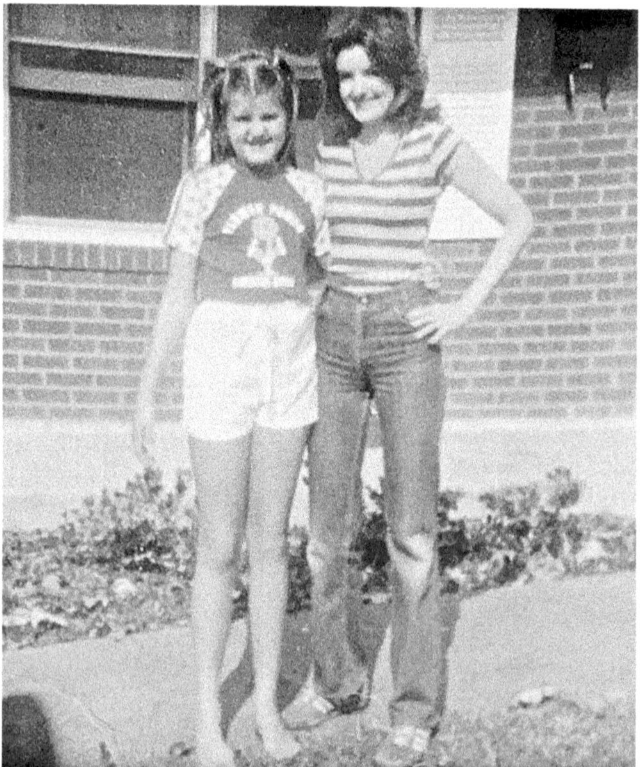

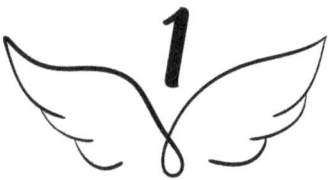

Discovering a Love for Fitness-Thanks, Mamma!

*M*y first memory of being in a gym was in junior high school. My mamma went to The Gym in our neighborhood, and yes, that was really the name. It was like you would imagine—no frills and no women. I only remember a room full of free weights, some benches, mirrors, and a few machines. Imagine the vibe of the gym in the movie *Rocky* in 1980.

There was one machine I specifically remember. I stood on it, strapped a belt on, and flipped the switch. It shook and jigged me all over, making me giggle. Even as a kid, I didn't think it was actually doing anything.

Praise Through the Pain

Although I was a little pudgy, no one ever told me. Back in the late seventies/early eighties, we didn't talk about body image like we do today. Thank God we didn't have the internet, social media, or any of the pressures and noise that come with them. Life was simple. We played outside until our knees were stained green and our hands gritty from climbing trees and racing bikes down cracked sidewalks. Laughter echoed through the neighborhood as we chased each other under the fading sun surrounded by the familiar chorus of cicadas and distant lawnmowers.

When the streetlights flickered on, it was our unspoken signal—time to hustle home before our parents noticed we weren't there. Back then, discipline wasn't about timers or text messages. It was simple, understood, and woven into the rhythm of our days. Discipline was different!

One time, I lost track of the streetlights because I'd slipped into my friend Lulu's house to watch *Flipper*, a television show about a boy and his pet dolphin. We were sprawled out on the shag carpet, completely caught up in the adventure, when a knock suddenly echoed through the front door. I hadn't even noticed the sun had set. We scrambled to answer, and there stood my dad. He didn't have to say a word. His look said it all. I knew I was in trouble, and I never missed the streetlights again.

There were no video games or cell phones to distract us back then. We played kickball and pretended we were "the Fonz" from *Happy Days* or one of "Charlie's Angels" as we zipped around the neighborhood on our bikes and skateboards. Sometimes we'd ride to the corner gas station for candy, feeling so grown up. I even tried my first cigarette with my neighbor friend—and coughed up my lungs! I decided that was enough rebellion for one day.

We weren't perfect. We were just regular kids getting into mostly good, clean fun with a dash of mischief. Life was simple. We even rode our bikes to school.

I went to Flowers Elementary in Montgomery, Alabama, and I still have an old photo of me grinning next to my mom in that cute Flower Power T-shirt. I treasure that picture—not just for the memory but for what it represents. My mamma was my first and greatest cheerleader.

Fitness was a meaningful part of her life for many years. She wasn't just passionate about getting stronger. She lived it, eventually working as a gym manager and inspiring others with her dedication. I remember her studying a book by Rachel McLish, one of the first female bodybuilders. I still have that book, and when I hold it, I picture Mamma's hands turning the pages, eager to learn and grow.

Later, a difficult relationship pulled her away from the gym and lifestyle she loved. But the foundation she built—her strength, her example, and her encouragement—left a lasting mark on me.

Because of my mamma's influence, I feel like I have always loved exercise, although I wouldn't call myself an athlete. In seventh grade, I signed up for softball with my best friend. My main memory? Standing out in right field watching the ball come straight at me. My instincts kicked in: I ducked and used my glove like a helmet shielding my head. Why didn't I just turn the glove around and catch it? Makes me laugh!

At home, I had a basketball goal in the backyard, but my only teammate was my German Shepherd. I used to think the neighborhood boys made fun of me when they watched, but now I wonder if they just thought it was cool that my dog played basketball, too.

It wasn't until junior high that I discovered I was good at long distance running. I could go forever without getting tired. Then came cheerleading and the dance team, where I discovered joy in movement.

Later, in college, I started lifting weights at the gym just like my mom did. I realized I was following in her footsteps. I'm grateful we shared a love for health and strength, and I carry her spirit with me in everything I do as "The Fitness Angel."

I am here to share my story of how God used fitness and nutrition to bless me with the title, "The Fitness Angel." My name is Angel, which means "messenger," and I truly believe God has called me to be a messenger for faith, fitness, and health. My deepest desire is to glorify God because without Him, I would not be the person I am today—His daughter, made uniquely and perfectly imperfect, with a heart to praise HIM and help others on their fitness and health journeys.

We all have a story. You were created with purpose. God can use your unique and even "crazy" self to show others just how amazing our God is! Maybe, along the way, you'll even learn how to dance and praise the LORD through life's hard times. We all face trials, but we overcome by the blood of the Lamb and the word of our testimony (*Revelation 12:11*). My hope is that my journey will encourage you to find strength, faith, and joy in your own.

I hope you feel inspired to begin your health journey, or maybe even kick it up a notch! And please know I'm praying and rooting for you along the way.

Reflections

1) What good things did you learn from your childhood that are serving you today?

2) Have you found joy in movement?

3) Practice gratitude by journaling or saying them out loud.

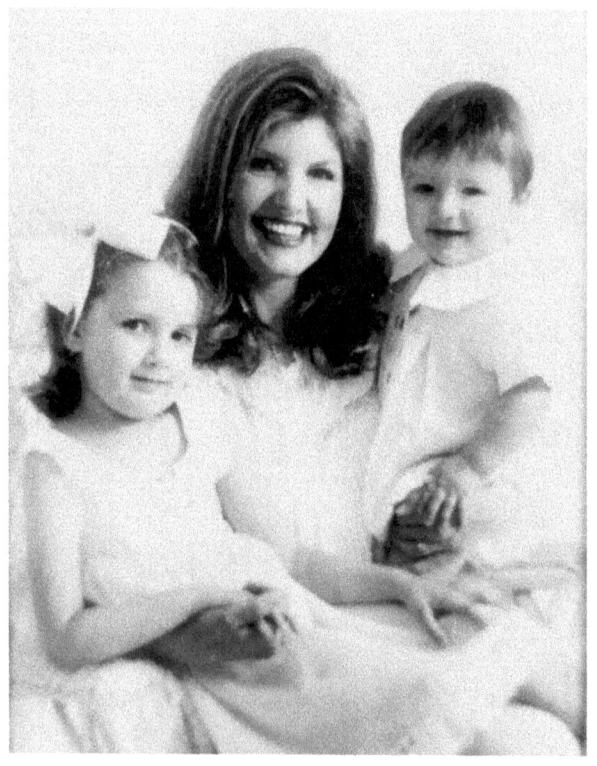

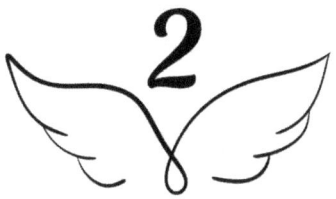

2

When Faith, Family, and Fitness Collide!

Now, at fifty-six, I love working out and teaching fitness classes. Walking is my favorite way to stay active. I could walk for hours, whether it's with our dogs, with my daughter Lydia, or just by myself. I never seem to get tired. Sometimes I listen to music or a podcast, but lately I've been prayer walking. Walking has become a huge part of my daily spiritual practice.

Often, I'll use the Lord's Prayer as my guide, breaking it apart and making it personal as I pour out my heart.

Here's an example.

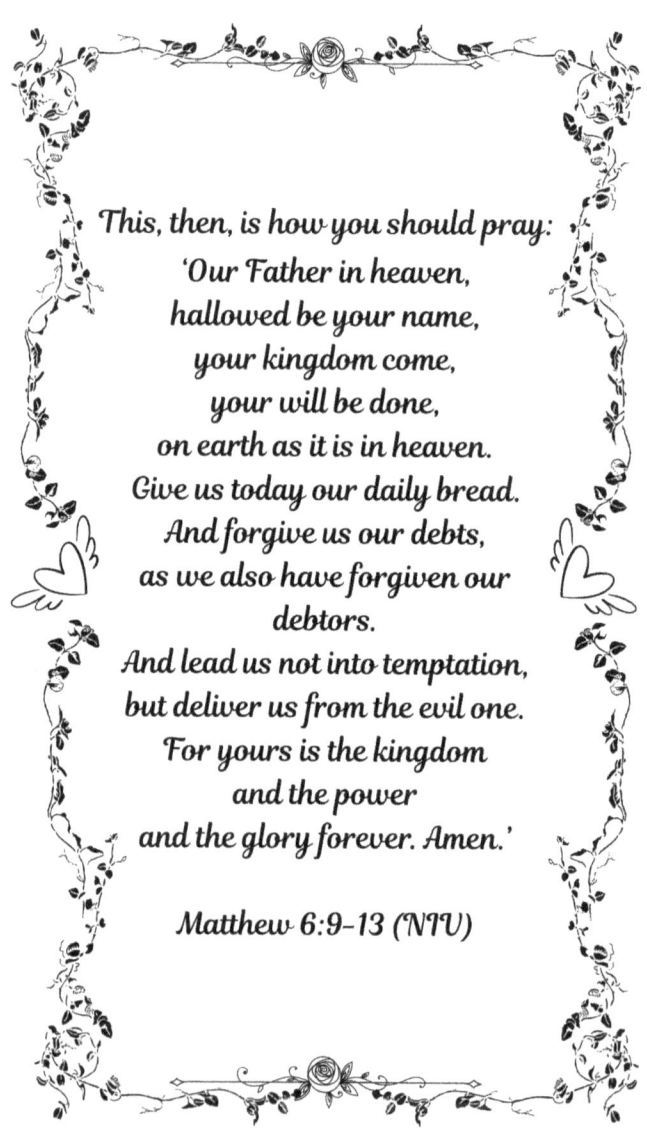

This, then, is how you should pray:
'Our Father in heaven,
hallowed be your name,
your kingdom come,
your will be done,
on earth as it is in heaven.
Give us today our daily bread.
And forgive us our debts,
as we also have forgiven our
debtors.
And lead us not into temptation,
but deliver us from the evil one.
For yours is the kingdom
and the power
and the glory forever. Amen.'

Matthew 6:9-13 (NIV)

- *Our Father, who art in Heaven, hallowed be thy name;* **(God, I praise you because you are HOLY! You are the one true God, and I worship you! Thank you for being my LORD! Thank you for sending Jesus to be my Savior! I give you all the glory!)**

- *Thy kingdom come; thy will be done, on earth as it is in Heaven.* **(I pray for Your will to be done! I pray for healing for my dear friends _____, _____, _____ in the name of Jesus! I pray for justice for my mamma. Let it be done on earth as it is done in Heaven.)**

- *Give us this day our daily bread.* **(Thank you for being my Provider! Thank you for supplying all my needs. Thank you for _____, _____, _____.)**

- *And forgive us our trespasses, as we forgive those who trespass against us.* **(Lord, I repent for _____. Please help me walk in forgiveness with _____, _____, and _____. Help me to be free from bitterness and anger at the wrongs done to me.**

- *And lead us not into temptation, but deliver us from the evil one. For thine is the kingdom, the power, and the glory, forever and ever. Amen.* **(Thank you, LORD, for your protection and covering. You are my shield! Help me keep my eyes on you and praise you all day long! I give you all the glory for every blessing and for your protection!)**

Praying God's Word with intention brings such clarity. Before I know it, I've walked over an hour and reached my goal of ten thousand steps!

Another way I love to prayer walk is by using the acronym PRAY, something I learned from my pastor:

> **P - PRAISE!** Start your walk with gratitude and thankfulness. Sometimes I'll start singing, "This is the day the LORD has made! I will rejoice and be glad in it!" Or I'll start thanking God for different things: thank you for the blue skies, thank you for the birds, thank you for this sunny day. Thank you for my husband who works so hard to provide for our family. Thank you for my health and that I can teach my classes. Thank you for my children who call me nearly every day. Thank you … you get the idea. The more you start thanking God, the more grateful you become, and the joy starts overflowing!

R - REPENT! This one is hard but necessary. The LORD says to confess your sins and be forgiven. Of course, we are saved by grace, but the quicker we can confess our sins, the better! Admit it, quit it, and forget it. Sometimes I'll sing, "Create in me a clean heart, O God, and renew a right spirit in me!" I love quoting Scripture and singing it! We can go straight to Jesus, our Great High Priest. He is faithful and just to forgive us. We can walk more joyfully knowing we have confessed our sins!

A - ASK! God wants us to ask for what we want. Our Father loves us and wants to give us good gifts. I like to ask in detail. The more detailed, the better. Create a vision of what you want; God already knows. He will put those desires in you as you delight in Him. Have a conversation with God asking Him to show you more details. This should put a smile on your face and fill you with excitement and expectation. This is how you build your faith muscles!

Y - YIELD! Surrender those dreams and desires to God. We must trust in His Will, His Way, and His Timing! If He wants it, we must trust it's going to happen. And if there are any desires not from Him, we ask those desires to go away. We must exhibit simple, child-like faith.

In addition to spending time with our Heavenly Father and taking care of our bodies as the temple He gave us, there are so many benefits to walking, especially as we age! First, it's free and simple. If it's raining outside, you can walk on a treadmill or walk around your house while watching walking workouts or listening to music or a podcast. You can even include shopping to help you get in those steps. Staying active is what matters!

In addition to walking, I love dancing. In junior high school, I tried out for cheerleading and made the team, but I struggled with the gymnastics part. Although I enjoyed being a cheerleader, I never felt like I fit in, and I didn't feel good enough. The next year when I didn't make the team, I tried out for the dance team and made it. I discovered I had a natural talent for dance, and I loved making up routines and practicing. When "The Eye of the Tiger" comes on today, I still remember that dance routine! Now when I'm teaching dance fitness classes or leading "Praise Parties" at churches, it feels like I'm leading a dance team. I get so much energy because I am my most authentic self. I love to feel the music, and I enjoy choreographing routines to Christian music. The lyrics strengthen my spirit and nurture my soul.

During college, I joined my first gym, Living Well Fitness Center, right by the bank where I worked. I walked in and signed up with my own money. Looking back, that felt like a big deal for me as a college student juggling multiple jobs to put myself through school. I was growing weary of the party scene and starting to seek God and the deeper meaning of life. Because I loved the energy of the gym, I traded time in the nightclubs for the gym.

Working out with the big guys, slinging heavy weights as my belt braced my back and gloves kept blisters at bay, then leaping straight into high-impact, Jane Fonda-inspired aerobics left me absolutely hooked! The rush of endorphins was incredible—I got into the best shape of my life: tiny, toned, fit, tan, and overflowing with unstoppable energy.

Majoring in education didn't exactly fill my college schedule with lively electives, so you can imagine my excitement when I spotted aerobics on the course list! I pounced on the chance to earn credit by working out. Charging through those classes, pushing my heart rate sky-high, breaking a sweat, and feeling that exhilarating burst of energy—exercise became my addiction. Nothing made me feel more alive than getting in those workouts!

At the time, my Aunt Kathy was reading a book called *Fit for Life*, promoting good nutrition. I tried it and felt great! I trusted my Aunt Kathy, Mamma's youngest sister, who loved me and taught me all my cheerleading skills. I'm so grateful for all the time she poured into me. I knew she believed in me and wanted the best for me.

While experiencing my physical body having a transformation with exercise and diet, my spirit hungered for more, too. It's amazing how our body, spirit, and soul are connected. I was developing a desire to understand God better. My dad's second wife gave me a New Living Translation Bible, so easy to read and understand. I began reading it on my own.

Around that same time, God sent an angel into my life, Ms. Geraldine Lee, a sweet and classy older lady I met while working at the bank. I had the honor of helping her with her account, and she invited me to church, even asking me to sit with her and her family. Ms. Lee recognized my hunger to know the LORD, and we became close, often talking about God, His Word, and His character. Although I hadn't fully surrendered my life to God, He was loving me and revealing wonderful truths through His Word. I even volunteered to teach Sunday school with a friend I invited to church—JoAnn, who was a little older than me. We'd go out on Saturday nights, then wake up for church on Sunday morning to teach first grade Sunday school. God was so patient with us! I know HE saw who we truly were, even before we did. It was a process, and through it, God taught me to be patient with others, too.

After graduating with a degree in education, there were no jobs to be found. It was a bad time in the economy; there was a hiring freeze, and teachers even had to supply their own toilet paper! I applied to teach at a Girl Scout camp for the summer where I would live in a tent with my poodle, Precious. Hesitantly, I accepted the position. But God had another plan.

I met my husband, Wade, at Auburn University at Montgomery (AUM), but he transferred to the main campus for pharmacy school. Then he moved to Pensacola, Florida, for his internship. I was jealous! Girl Scout camp or the beach? As a free spirit, I didn't hesitate to pack up a U-Haul and my poodle and go to the beach! I wasn't thinking long term … I just wanted to live at the beach for a while.

Little did I know, God was setting me up for something BIG! I quickly got a full-time job at

Parisian department store in the mall. I also joined a local gym that had a ladies-only section. You could find me at the six o'clock step aerobics class every morning. I honestly felt addicted, and Wade said I even did aerobics in my sleep!

As we both searched for more than just a mundane life, we discovered Brownsville Assembly of God Church. The pastor taught sermons with boldness and authority. Hungry for God's truths, we went Sunday morning, Sunday night, and Wednesday night.

One evening after church, Wade needed to stop by the hospital to pick up some paperwork for school. I waited outside in his green convertible, the parking lot almost completely silent—no cars, no voices, just calm. The air was warm with a gentle breeze, and I felt an overwhelming sense of peace settle over me.

That's when it happened: I heard God speak to me for the very first time. It wasn't an out loud voice, but it was something clear and unmistakable—quiet, but powerful—right in my mind and deep in my heart. I sensed Him saying, "Now is the time." Instantly, I understood what that meant. It was time to surrender my life to Jesus.

Right there, sitting in that parked car, I bowed my head and whispered a simple prayer. "Lord, I surrender my heart to You. I don't want to live for myself anymore. Come live inside of me and take over my life." At that moment, I was born again. Jesus saved me, and I've never looked back.

Three months later, Wade and I married. We loved Pensacola, the sunshine, seafood, beach, and warm air, but were eager for him to graduate and for us to start our family. We moved to Auburn, Alabama, where Wade finished pharmacy school. There, we attended Auburn First Assembly of God Church where I was baptized in the Holy Spirit and filled with His Power!

I became a Holy Spirit-filled preaching machine everywhere I went. I worked at the bank, joined Gold's Gym, and worked out every day; I loved sharing the gospel with every person I met. I was truly on fire for God, and I feel the same today!

I'm endlessly grateful that our little church taught us the power of praise. Praising God—even before the miracle comes—became a life lesson I've clung to through every season, especially the toughest ones! Praise is not just thanksgiving—it's spiritual warfare. God knew I would need this weapon in the battles that lay ahead.

Dancing before the Lord became an essential part of my journey, a way to celebrate, pour out my thankfulness, and lay my heart wide open—sometimes with laughter, sometimes with tears streaming down my face. In those moments, I discover fresh freedom and joy. Praise transforms even the hardest days, turning weakness into strength and despair into hope. Here are some of my favorite verses where dancing was an act of worship and celebration:

"Let them praise his name with dancing and make music to him with timbrel and harp."
Psalm 149:3, NIV

"You turned my wailing into dancing; you removed my sackcloth and clothed me with joy."
Psalm 30:11, NIV

"Wearing a linen ephod, David was dancing before the Lord with all his might."
2 Samuel 6:14, NIV

Praise isn't just something I do—it's a spiritual lifeline and a weapon of warfare. When I choose to praise God, especially in the middle of difficulties or spiritual attacks, I'm actively resisting the enemy and aligning my heart with the truth of who God is. Praise silences fear, breaks through anxiety, and pushes back the darkness. It confuses the enemy and reminds my soul who's in control. And God makes miracles happen!

> *"About midnight Paul and Silas were praying and singing hymns to God, and the other prisoners were listening to them. Suddenly there was such a violent earthquake that the foundations of the prison were shaken. At once all the prison doors flew open, and everyone's chains came loose."*
> Acts 16:25-26, NIV

After those transformative lessons in praise and worship, a new chapter opened for us. Once Wade graduated, he landed his first pharmacy job in the tiny town of Enterprise, Alabama. Suddenly, we found ourselves close to family and just a quick trip from the beach. I started teaching at a

Christian school, we threw ourselves into church life, and I even ran children's camps at the YMCA. It was a sweet season—simple, full of purpose, and knit together by faith.

But deep in my heart, I longed for more: to become a mom and to one day live in a city bustling with opportunity. Those dreams led us back to Montgomery, where I taught at Evangel Christian Academy, our favorite church's school. Looking back, that season overflowed with growth. So much of God's Word came alive in me. My daily prayer walks through our neighborhood became my only exercise, yet I was content and grateful for those quiet, sacred moments.

Not long after, the answer to one of my prayers came: I became pregnant with a baby boy. But at Christmas time, heartbreak stuck—he passed away in my womb. It was my first true devastation as a believer. The pain was raw and confusing, and I found myself wrestling deeply with God, starting to learn what it means to walk with Him through suffering.

> *"Dear friends, so do not be surprised*
> *at the fiery ordeal that has come on*
> *you to test you, as though*
> *something strange were happening*
> *to you. But rejoice inasmuch as you*
> *participate in the sufferings of Christ,*
> *so that you may be overjoyed when*
> *His glory is revealed."*
> 1 Peter 4:12-13, NIV

After losing our baby, my heart broke in ways I never expected. That deep loss reshaped me, opening my eyes and heart to the value of every life, and it's what led me to become passionately pro-life and serve as a counselor at a crisis pregnancy center. Walking with other women through their own crossroads gave a sense of purpose to my pain—I could remind them their stories weren't over, even if they couldn't see it yet.

But healing is often layered. My own journey with infertility soon followed. Month after month, hope seemed just out of reach, and sometimes the doubts felt heavier than my faith. I'll never forget a conversation in the ladies room at church: A woman, older and well-meaning, gently told me that Wade and I were already a complete family, even if children never came. Her words stung. She meant to comfort me, but in my heart, I knew I couldn't let her perspective shape my faith.

That's when I learned that sometimes praise is the boldest act of faith. Instead of giving in to despair, I chose to worship. Week after week in church, I would lift my Bible high during worship and proclaim, "Whose report will you believe? We shall believe the report of the Lord!" With every song and every prayer, I reminded my soul that God's promises are true, even when my circumstances disagreed. Praise became more than music—it became my lifeline, building up my faith when hope ran low and helping me silence the voices of doubt, both inside and out.

During that season of waiting and worship, Philippians 4:6-7 became a lifeline to me: *"Do not be anxious about anything, but in every situation, by prayer and petition, with thanksgiving, present your requests to God. And the peace of God, which transcends all understanding, will guard your hearts and your minds in Christ Jesus"* (NIV).

That verse stopped me in my tracks. I remember reading it and looking up the word petition. What I found moved me deeply—it meant "a formal written request made to a king." That's when something shifted in my spirit. God wasn't just listening passively. He was reigning sovereignly, and I could come boldly before Him as His daughter, with my heart's deepest desire.

In the blank space right next to that verse in my Bible, I wrote out my petition to the King of kings. The date was May 13, 1996. I wrote:

I am petitioning God for a healthy pregnancy, birth, and most importantly, a healthy baby. I will continue to pray with thanksgiving, believing that God my Father, will give me the desires of my heart.

Your daughter,
Angel Faulk.

Exactly one year and one day later, on May 14, 1997, at 3:59 p.m., that prayer was answered. I held in my arms a healthy baby girl—Lydia Marie Faulk. And right there in my Bible next to that petition, I wrote these two simple, victorious words: "Answered Prayer."

Becoming a stay-at-home mom was a dream come true. I threw myself into church and Bible study and poured my heart into being a mom. My daily walks with the stroller became my favorite exercise—simple joys, a soul at peace.

Everything changed when a friend invited me to her gym. I wanted to join, but it wasn't in our budget. So I got creative: Why not work there part-time and earn a free membership? I started by folding towels and checking in members.

God's timing is always spot on. About a month in, the manager pulled me aside and declared, "You should be teaching classes!" I was blown away. I'd always loved jumping in with every class—step aerobics, spin, you name it— and suddenly the door was wide open. Confidence kicked in: I can do this! Even better, a national fitness certification training landed at our local university. I signed up, full of butterflies and expectation.

That was nearly thirty years ago, and I've been teaching fitness classes ever since! From the start, I have woven my faith into every class— playing Christian music and sharing Scripture or nuggets from my morning quiet time. Most mornings, I'd head straight from my Bible and prayer into the studio, overflowing with hope and encouragement to give away. It felt natural and right. I was simply being myself.

But sometimes God redirects our steps in ways we never expect. One morning, after teaching class, I walked in to pick up baby Lydia from the gym's nursery only to find the worker pinching her. Shocked and heartbroken, I stood up for my daughter, reported what I'd seen, and when my boss sided with the worker, I quit on the spot. I held Lydia close and left … tears in my eyes but peace in my heart.

Driving straight to the YMCA, I told the manager my story, auditioned the same day, and was hired on the spot. For over twenty years, the YMCA became my home, letting me teach all kinds of classes, earn multiple certifications, and grow in ways I never imagined. It's an organization that truly supports body, mind, and spirit. Not only did they allow me to play Christian music, I was able to pray with members and even lead Bible studies. Members often told me they loved my classes and felt like they "had church" after class. It's where my passion for faith and fitness truly took flight.

If there's anything I've learned, it's this: when God closes a door, He always has something better in store! Looking back, every twist and turn has somehow woven together faith, family, health, and purpose—not just for me, but for my children, too. That's how "The Fitness Angel" was born: through God's guidance, a mother's heart, and a passion to help others find strength in body and spirit.

Just as life with Lydia felt like a miracle, another incredible blessing was on its way—our son, Ethan. Lydia was only two, but my heart bubbled over with excitement to be pregnant again. The Lord answered our prayers before we even knew to ask!

Before we discovered his gender, a dear friend who was gifted in prophecy told me, "You'll have a boy. He'll be tall, dark, and handsome, and he'll lead many to the Lord. He's going to be a prophet!" Her words filled me with hope and expectation.

As I reached six months, I realized I wasn't growing as much as I should have been, and at my appointment, the doctor showed concern. Fear tried to press in—especially since we'd lost our first son, John David, at five months. I was admitted to the hospital for testing, my faith stretched thin as I waited for answers. Relief and gratitude washed over me when they found his heartbeat strong, and I could feel Ethan wiggling, a reminder that God was still writing this story.

Once home, I longed for community and support, so I slipped out of Lydia's usual children's class at church where I volunteered and into a prayer meeting. When I shared my heart, friends gathered around, praying with power and compassion. Someone else spoke of a vision of our son as a prophet—confirmation of Ethan's destiny. Together, we waged spiritual warfare—praying, praising, and boldly proclaiming God's purpose for Ethan even before he entered the world.

Name searches in our family always come back to the Bible. "Ethan" means strong—and Ethan in Scripture was a worship leader. "Samuel" was a prophet and a testimony to answered prayer. So we named him Ethan Samuel—a declaration of strength, worship, and prophetic destiny.

Years later, when Ethan discovered his love for drums, he found his name in 2 Chronicles as one who played cymbals in worship. The threads of prophecy, his gifts, and God's Word all wove together, just as God had spoken through my friend, Debra, long before we ever knew he'd be a boy. And sure enough, he grew up tall, dark, and handsome, with a spirit of worship and a heart called to God.

Ethan's story serves as a living reminder that God's plans for our children are bigger, better, and more miraculous than we could ever dream and that His promises, spoken over us in faith, never return void.

As I prayed over Ethan and trusted God through every twist and turn of his life, the Lord gave me a verse that leaked it all in my heart:

> *"For I know the plans I have for you, declares the Lord, "plans to prosper you and not to harm you, plans to give you hope and a future."*
> Jeremiah 29:11, NIV

That promise has never left me. It was true when I carried him in faith, just as it's true now as I watch him grow into everything God created him to be.

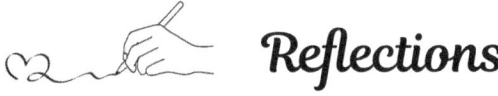 *Reflections*

1) Did you have someone encourage you as a child, like my aunt poured into me? Stop and thank God for that person.

2) Reflect on when God was patient with you, similar to when I was a young adult, not yet a born again Christian, partying on Saturday night and teaching Sunday school. Who do you need to be more patient with?

3) When God closes a door, He has something better, although it requires faith. Journal about a time God closed and opened doors for you. Did you exercise faith or anxiety and fear?

4) Have you experienced the power of praise? What is your favorite way to praise the Lord?

5) Are you a mother? Has God written big plans for your children in your heart?

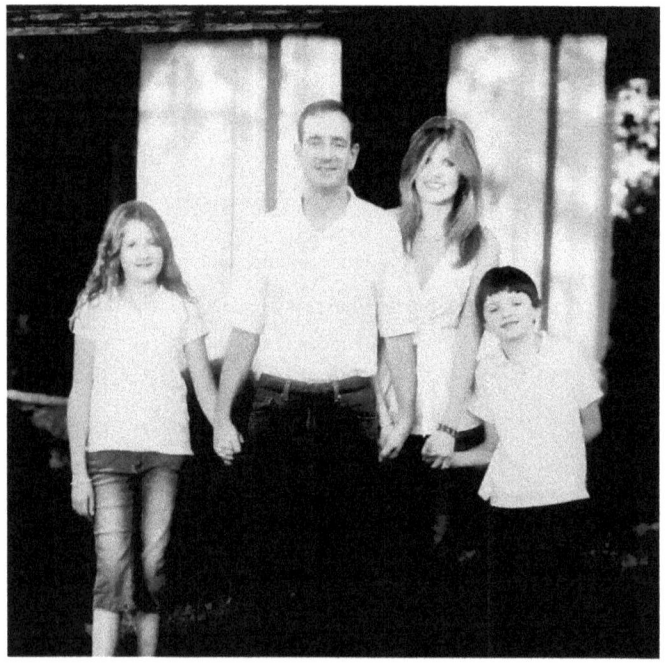

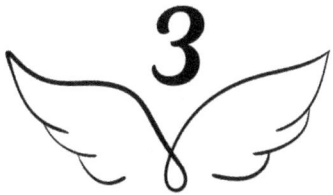

Moving to Tennessee—The Best Decision

*T*hroughout my spiritual journey, I've learned that God often weaves the good with the bad, yet His timing is always perfect. While still in Montgomery, Wade played guitar on our church worship team, and I continued to teach at "the Y" and serve in children's ministry. Lydia was four, and our son, Ethan, had just turned one. Life seemed perfect!

That's when the worst tragedy imaginable occurred. I'll share the story in another book, but the trauma was too much to handle. We felt so devastated that we couldn't bear to live in the same environment. That's when we moved to

Franklin, Tennessee, for a fresh start in life and new surroundings. I couldn't take the triggers I was dealing with daily in Montgomery.

Near Nashville, Franklin had been voted the best place to raise a family in the South, so we felt good about the decision. Wade loved playing guitar, and we both especially loved Christian music. While in Montgomery, we had made friends with a couple who moved to Franklin around the same time to start a music career. Chris and Wade had played on the worship team in our Montgomery church, so imagine our excitement to have close friends with small children close to our children's ages in our new hometown. We started going to the same church. Wade and Chris played together again in the worship band. Leah and I volunteered in children's ministry together and were involved in women's ministry and Bible study. We did everything together. Wade quickly found a wonderful pharmacy job. I told the realtor I wanted to live near the YMCA. God blessed us with the sweetest home—a place where we would raise our children and spend the next twenty years. It felt like we were living in the fictitious television town, Mayberry. Our house was just down the road from the Franklin YMCA, nestled in a charming, tree-lined neighborhood.

The same weekend we moved in, I walked into the YMCA, applied to become a substitute fitness instructor, and started teaching fitness classes almost immediately. Before long, I had my own classes and taught nearly every day, even at other local gyms. But "the Y" truly became like family.

The same group of women attended my classes for two decades. Together, we took turns leading Bible studies and grew spiritually as well as physically. Scripture adorned the walls, and a large Bible sat open on a podium at the entrance to the group fitness room. Everyone knew this was a godly place. I was even invited to join the

Spirit Board, where I helped encourage spiritual growth among the members. I thank God every day for my time at "the Y." That community became my family, especially when I faced a frightening diagnosis—a brain tumor that changed my life forever!

It started with hearing loss in 2006. I began losing the ability to hear on my right side, and I went to the doctor for a hearing test. I thought it would be a simple visit. In my mind, I had decided it was due to too much loud music in my fitness classes. We were always told to "turn it down," but for some reason we always felt more energy with the music UP! To my surprise, the ear, nose, and throat doctor (ENT) told me I did have hearing loss, but it wasn't from loud music. He had no other explanation. I was told to "keep an eye on it" and to let him know if it got worse.

I should have asked more questions and dug deeper. I wonder how many busy moms overlook their own health issues because they are too busy taking care of everybody else. This is a lesson I hope you receive. Take care of YOU! Your body is the temple of the Holy Spirit. Your body is your home on this earth, and if you don't take care of it, you will not be able to care for your family. If something isn't right, there is a reason. We must keep looking until we find answers. To this day, I want to blame the doctor for not having been more proactive. This experience taught me to be a better advocate for myself and my health.

Things did get worse, very gradually. I started using my left ear to talk on the phone. I started asking everyone to repeat themselves because I couldn't hear unless I leaned my left ear in a little closer.

Three years after that initial visit for a hearing test I was in for a shock!

I was sound asleep in the middle of the night when I was awakened with a loud, crunching sound inside my right ear. It sounded as if someone was crushing paper. Then

SILENCE. I jumped out of bed, ran to the bathroom, and looked in the mirror to see what was happening to my ear. Of course there was no change in appearance. When I put my finger over my ear to test the hearing, hoping for something, I got nothing. I was 100 percent deaf on the right side. This was so scary!

I called the doctor's office as soon as it opened, and they got me in immediately. My doctor was also my neighbor and friend, Dr. Jeff Suppinger. After a full examination and not seeing anything, he suggested I go back to the ENT. They worked me in. Unfortunately, he confirmed I had lost all hearing on the right side and suggested an MRI. Since I was going to California the next day to visit family for seven days, the doctor told me it was not urgent and to enjoy my vacation, but to get the MRI when I returned home.

Not knowing why I had this hearing loss made it a difficult trip for those seven days. I still enjoyed myself. I am blessed that God made me a joyful person, full of faith, and always having fun. But I admit I was concerned, and it stayed on my mind. We made jokes that "Mom can't hear!" I am so grateful I knew 2 Timothy 1:7, that *"God has not given me a spirit of fear, but of love, power, and a sound mind."* I knew I could always trust God, no matter what. Even if it meant there would be suffering involved.

When I returned from our trip, I ended up having to schedule my own MRI because the doctor's office forgot. I was learning again that I had to become my own health advocate. We cannot depend on anybody else! Unfortunately, Wade had to work that day, a Friday afternoon, probably the worst time for an important appointment. It means waiting over the weekend before getting test results, and waiting is the hardest. But being an optimist, I made a decision not to worry. I put my hope in God, believing it would be okay.

I drove my minivan to the medical office, which oddly enough was across the street from the ENT's office. As I parked my van, I could see the ENT office building and was reminded once again of the unknown. If you've ever had a medical issue, I'm sure you can relate. So many emotions can trigger fear and uncertainty. That's when being in constant conversation with God is especially important. When we know God's Word and His character, we know we can trust Him no matter what, even if it's scary.

I went inside the office, and it was packed. After signing in, I found an empty chair and began the waiting process. I looked around at all the faces and wondered what their stories were. I knew each person there had a story, and many were in fear. I could see it on their faces, burdened with the cares of the world.

Finally, I was called back. The nurse guided me to a changing room with a locker and told me where to wait after changing. Posters covered the walls—posters of brain tumors! My first thought was NO WAY am I having a brain tumor. Then the thought hit me, "What if?"

I was a fitness instructor, a picture of perfect health. I'd never been seriously sick. Of course, I had seasonal allergies and occasional colds, but nothing serious. How could this be happening?

Once I was taken to the MRI room, I was given directions to lay on the machine. It was so cold! They gave me a thin blanket, but I still shivered. The technician got me another blanket. He was very calm and compassionate and wanted me to be comfortable. He gave me an emergency cord to hold and told me to squeeze it at any time I needed to come out of the MRI machine. This was a forty-five-minute MRI, and after being rolled inside, I understood how it could be difficult for a claustrophobic person. Thankfully, I do not struggle with that.

I was told to be perfectly still so they could get an accurate reading. It was easy for me because he gave me headphones and folded towels around me to keep my head from moving. Halfway through the test, they injected me with Gadolinium to highlight any abnormalities. It felt strange shooting through my veins. Later I read it could cause paralysis. Glad I didn't know that beforehand. I survived the test, and when it was over, I realized I had been at the appointment for hours. It was getting dark outside.

After getting dressed and ready to leave, I realized I was the last patient. I noticed a hallway office door ajar and saw my technician looking at a brain scan on his desk. I knew it had to be mine. I asked him if I could see it. He looked shocked that I would ask. He had a sad look on his face and nodded slowly.

I walked closer and saw the brain … my brain. The left side was perfectly normal; however, the right side was almost completely mashed by a HUGE tumor! I was in disbelief, stunned. I looked into the technician's eyes and the words slowly came out, "I have a brain tumor?"

He slowly nodded his head, confirming this inconceivable news. He had a computer disk with all the information. I told him I wanted to take it home to show my husband. He said I couldn't have it, and I'd have to meet with the doctor. He confessed he wasn't supposed to share this news with me and that the disks were nearly impossible to understand unless you were trained to read thio particular scan, I told him my pharmacist husband was brilliant, and he could figure it out. He hesitantly agreed and gave me the disk.

I quickly took it before he could change his mind and raced to my van as if I were escaping this nightmare before it could even begin. I got into my van and looked around. I was so angry as I gazed across the parking lot at the ENT office. Three years ago, I had known something was wrong, but felt dismissed, as if my life didn't matter. I wanted to march into that office and let them know how I felt! Of course, every medical office was closed.

I couldn't help but notice the restaurant across from me where beautiful families celebrated the weekend. I was reminded of my precious family—my husband and our children. Lydia was twelve years old, my mini me! We were homeschooling and did everything together. She was active in singing, piano, acting, and Girl Scouts. We were always going to meetings, practices, plays, and church events. Ethan was nine years old, smart and super social. He also took piano, but preferred basketball, playing with neighborhood friends, biking, and building Legos. My kids were everything to me. My world centered on being a wife and mom. How would this affect their lives? How would things change? What about my fitness classes? How would my life change? All these thoughts flooded my mind.

I called Wade, who worked as a pharmacist at the busiest CVS Pharmacy in the Nashville area. He never had his phone on or nearby. I only called during an emergency. Since he knew where I was, he answered right away, knowing it must be important. I couldn't hold back my tears when I told him I had a brain tumor. He immediately said, "It will be okay." And I believed him.

We had weathered many storms together. I knew God had gotten us through everything in the past, and He was faithful! God would get us through this, too!

I got home and waited for him. He closed the store and arrived home by ten o'clock. We stayed up until midnight, looking at the scan, and looking online to learn what type of brain tumor I had and the possible treatments. I was proud of my brilliant husband—I knew I was right when I told the technician to give me the scan! We continued to pray in faith and believed God for my healing, even if it meant we had a treacherous journey ahead. We knew we could do anything with strength from our God!

We waited patiently all weekend and finally went to the ENT on Monday so he could tell us more. We had so many questions. What will the next steps be? Surgery? When and with whom and where? What would the possible outcome be, and what will recovery look like? What type of tumor is this?

Disappointment came when the doctor nonchalantly walked into the room. He smiled as if he was clueless! He didn't even know why we were there. He didn't seem to remember me. I cried quietly with a tissue in my hand. After his inappropriate greeting and our cold return, he apparently knew something was not right. He looked at my chart and exclaimed, "Oh, I see you had an MRI."

I couldn't remain quiet anymore. I yelled, "Yes, I did! I have a brain tumor!" I wanted to say,

"YOU IDIOT!" But the Holy Spirit kept me quiet. He realized his mistake and apologized. He then explained I should see Dr. David Haynes, a surgeon who understood these types of tumors and could schedule a surgery with me. We left the office and NEVER heard from him again! I'm sure he realized his negligence.

We scheduled an appointment with Dr. Haynes and were hopeful he had answers. Going into his office was like starting over. Another hearing test revealed I didn't have hearing on the right side. Then we met Dr. Haynes, a caring, compassionate, and confident man, his coffee in hand. He immediately brought calmness. He invited a group of medical students to join our appointment with our permission. They ran me through a series of balance and coordination exercises. They were amazed at what I could do. I explained I had been teaching fitness classes for twelve years, and the only issue I had was hearing.

The students left the room, leaving Wade, Dr. Haynes, and me. Dr. Haynes began to explain the tumor. He was concerned because the tumor had tails intertwining the nerves on the brain stem.

He said they had to be so careful as he intertwined his fingers together to show how delicate the surgery would be, like a game of pickup sticks! That's when I noticed he was missing digits! He literally was missing fingers, and I couldn't hear anything after that. It was like Charlie Brown's teacher talking. His words were coming out, and he was moving his mouth, but all I could hear was "waaa, waaa, waaa." I thought there was no way he could operate on my brain!

When he left the room to get his nurse so she could discuss scheduling, Wade and I just stared at each other in disbelief. The nurse came in, and we asked her HOW he could be a brain surgeon. She laughed and said everyone thinks that at first. She then explained his credentials and background, and we developed a peace and calm.

Soon after, Dr. Haynes rejoined us in the room. He explained this surgery would be very long, and he would invite his colleague, Dr. Reid Thompson, to partner with him in the surgery. Our next step was to meet Dr. Thompson. We scheduled that appointment next. This was the beginning of a lot of appointments!

Meeting Dr. Thompson was a different kind of experience. They are both fabulous surgeons but have very different personalities. While Dr. Haynes and his office were calm and his students had that same calmness, Dr. Thompson was animated and charismatic, his office busy and more crowded. It was more like the serious business of brain surgery. His students seemed on "high alert" when Dr. Thompson showed me the MRI, revealing this devilish design of the tumor. But he, just like Dr. Haynes, seemed perfectly confident that we could get the tumor out and save my life.

The tumor was benign, but its location was fatal, and it had to come out. I was thankful for the hearing loss after it crushed my auditory nerve. Sadly, others who have this tumor don't have symptoms or don't take them seriously, and they die in their sleep!

Dr. Thompson warned me the surgery would be extremely long and gruesome, but he believed I would live and be back to life as normal within one and a half years! I was an extremely active fitness instructor, wife, and mom. I loved my energetic life, and I needed to prepare for a long road to recovery, he said. BUT GOD had a different plan!

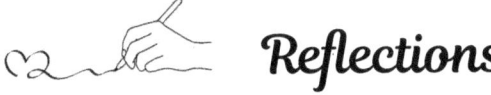 *Reflections*

1) Recall a time when God sent you a message that something wasn't quite right. Did you pay attention to the "nudging" or did you dismiss it? Take time to reflect on what you learned from that experience and allow it to strengthen your relationship with God.

2) Has God gotten you or a loved one through a difficult diagnosis? Journal about that time period and look for the hidden blessings.

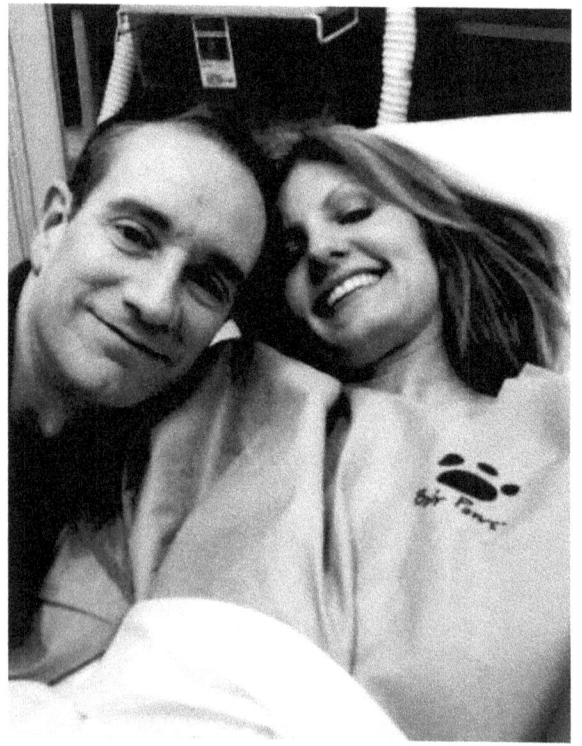

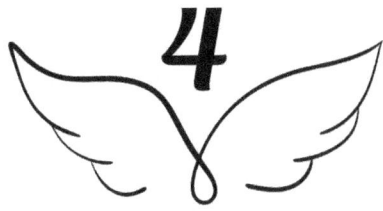

Touched by an Angel!

In the days leading up to my diagnosis and the daunting prospect of life-altering brain surgery, the only place I wanted to be was at Bible study. Something deep within urged me to go—to surrender my fear, to offer my heart and soul to God, and to ask for His complete healing. I needed Him to be with me every step of the way, knowing how uncertain life felt with such a surgery looming.

Despite everything, I carried that mustard seed faith—a quiet assurance that I would be okay, even if it was only deep down. At the Bible study I was attending, my friend Denise

Hildreth led our group through the book of Hebrews. We began, as always, with praise and worship. Drawn to the altar, I listened as our anointed worship leader, Tina Keil, sang my new favorite song, "Healer" by Kari Jobe. Not long before, someone—still unknown—had left the CD in my mailbox. Perhaps it was an angel; I certainly believe it was someone sent by God. That song played on repeat in my car, and now Tina was singing it right there at Bible study. I knew the Lord was blessing me in the midst of my fear. In those sacred moments at the altar, I closed my eyes in worship and heard God speak quietly to my heart:

First: *"You will be pleasantly surprised."*

Second: *"Your faith has made you whole."*

I recognized the scripture from Mark 5:34, where Jesus, speaking to the woman healed by her faith, said, *"Daughter, your faith has healed you. Go in peace and be freed from your suffering."* I didn't know what "pleasantly surprised" would be, but I remembered what I learned years before. God heals us in one of three ways: before the fire, after the fire, or by welcoming us home into His arms. Whatever the outcome of surgery—protection, process, or paradise—I trusted that God's healing would meet me.

My surgery was fourteen hours long, and the LORD was with us from the beginning. We even had a miraculous time just before surgery after checking in. When we arrived at Vanderbilt Hospital around 5:30 a.m., it was still dark outside. We did the paperwork, basically signing my life away. Then we gathered in the large waiting room. Our dear best friend, Edie Ross, and our life group leader from church, Doug Beiden, came to pray with us before going back. We sat and chatted and shared what the doctor said about the surgery and recovery. We noticed three other families gathered together, also waiting for their surgery. They had a small suitcase, pillow, and that same "concerned" look on their faces.

But there was one odd-looking lady sitting all alone—no purse, no suitcase, and no pillow. She had on jeans and a black hoodie. The hood was pulled down so I couldn't see her eyes. She was leaning back in her chair as if she was resting, her arms folded across her chest. Oddly, she smiled a big gorgeous smile, although I couldn't see her face or eyes due to the lighting and her position. It was as if she knew me.

She reminded me so much of my dear friend, Leah Walls, my best friend when we first moved to Franklin in 2003. Leah and her husband, Chris, were the ones who had moved from Montgomery close to the same time we did. After three years, they had moved to Arizona for a job change, and an unimaginable tragedy occurred. They were killed in a horrific car accident. Our lives were changed forever. Wade quit playing in the worship band and eventually wanted to change churches. He had a deep sadness and wouldn't talk about it. He has never had a friend since. It's as if he didn't want to experience that pain again.

That morning in the waiting room, as we stood and held hands in a circle and began to pray, our "friend in the black hoodie" rose from her chair. Wade noticed she stood behind me as we prayed. It's as if she was invisible to everyone in the room except Wade and me. After we prayed and opened our eyes, she had vanished! Was she an angel? Was it Leah? Only God knows! It wasn't any type of thing we prayed for or asked for, but we believe God did it!

"Do not neglect to show hospitality to strangers, for by so doing some have entertained angels without knowing it."
Hebrews 13:2 (NIV)

After praying, we were called back to the surgery area. After getting in a gown, I was wheeled into a room where I met all the attending nurses and anesthesiologists, and Dr. Haynes greeted me. He had a smile on his face, and I felt a peace that everything would go well. I asked if we could pray. Everyone agreed and bowed their heads. I was grateful and prayed for my healing and guidance over everyone involved. I had such a peace that God would be glorified through this challenge.

During the fourteen hours of surgery, Wade was never alone. Many friends came and visited throughout the day and night. Different women connected and met for the first time, becoming lifelong friends. Wade was truly blessed with their prayers, support, and encouragement. He had no clue how loved we were. The body of Christ was real, and he was experiencing it!

When I awoke to someone shaking my shoulder, I was in the middle of dreaming. I couldn't wait to tell Ethan. He asked if I thought I might dream during surgery. I also remembered that I had surgery and realized I was alive! I could think clearly, but I couldn't respond.

They took me to a room where I slept more. This time, I awoke to a room full of people, and they were cheering that I was okay. Wade looked so relieved. I guessed everything must have gone well. But I couldn't move my body, and I was covered in blankets. I was so hot. I couldn't take the blankets off, and I couldn't speak. Wade knew I wanted something, and he had the idea to help me write. He got a pencil and paper and held my hand. I tried with all my might to write the letters H-O-T but couldn't do it. I thought this must be what it feels like to be a child and all that pressure is on you, but the task is just too difficult.

Then something rose within me, and I tried again. This time Wade could read it and said out loud, "H-O-T. Angel is HOT!"

Edie said, "Yes she is!" Everyone laughed, but all I could think was, "These people are brilliant brain surgeons. Can't they take off my blankets?"

It's funny how the brain works. I could think so clearly, but the words wouldn't leave my mouth, and I couldn't move my body. How long was this recovery going to be, I wondered. I was determined to be strong and recover fast! I wanted to get my life back.

It took a few days, but I was eventually walking down the hall with a walker. The therapists said I should go to an outpatient hospital, but Dr. Thompson assured me I would be going home soon. His confidence encouraged my confidence and determination to grow.

One milestone I will never forget was going to the bathroom by myself. I had not looked in a mirror, but I knew I had facial paralysis. They said it would go away. Dr. Haynes said it would "hopefully" heal, but it was a possibility it wouldn't. I wanted to see my face. Once I made it to the bathroom, I had to muster up some courage before looking in the mirror. Then I did it. I saw my face, and immediately the Holy Spirit reminded me that I am an overcomer! I said, "Here we go LORD. Another adventure!" I knew HE had gotten me through some tough times, and I would get through this, too. When you belong to the LORD, you know you can do anything with HIM!

After three days, I went home. They said I had the healthiest heart they had ever seen in the intensive care unit. Teaching aerobics for twelve years had made an impact, and I was ready to get back to the gym, my classes, and my life!

Wade bought a shower chair, but I refused to use it. Our bedroom was upstairs, and somehow, I felt determined not to treat myself any differently, although I couldn't walk without assistance.

Ethan had been praying I could go trick or treating down our street. My surgery was October 21, so I had ten days. Wade and I walked up and down the street, and I was ready on October 31! Ethan ended up trick or treating with friends, and I sat on the front porch handing out candy. As I watched neighborhood kiddos on hayrides and neighbors dressed in costumes, tables covered with treats, I realized just how happy and blessed I was. Thank you, God!

Reflections

1) Mindset is everything! When has having a positive attitude helped you?

Write about it. Ask God if you need to shift your thinking in a particular area today.

2) Have you experienced an angel in your presence?

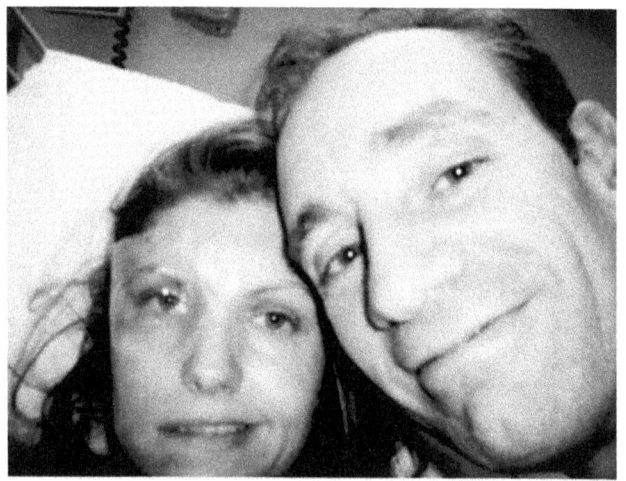

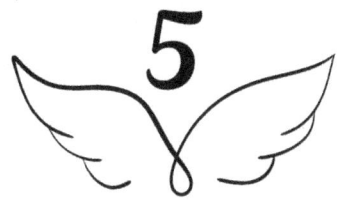

Facial Paralysis–
Harder Than Expected

I was healing and feeling better physically, but I forgot how I "looked" until a tween girl saw me Halloween night and screamed—she thought I was dressed up as a scary monster.

I had on my eye bubble, which was a clear shield to protect my eye from dryness since I was unable to blink or close it due to facial paralysis. Also, it had to be protected and kept moist. My head was shaved on one side with a huge scar that started next to my ear and went down my neck to my back. There was dried blood. I had on sweats with a huge blanket laying on my lap. For some reason, her scare surprisingly hurt my feelings, so I retreated inside and watched my all-time favorite movie, *ET*. I was reminded life wasn't "normal" and wouldn't be for a while, although I had hope I would heal completely.

In order to make that happen, I started every therapy available! Thankfully, Vanderbilt is a great hospital with excellent resources and comprehensive care. I had occupational therapy to make sure I could still write a grocery list. Thankfully, I passed with flying colors. I had speech therapy since the damaged facial nerve had affected my speech. Funny thing—my voice changed, too! My kids said I sounded like the *Wizard of Oz* munchkins.

Facial therapy aimed to restore strength in the affected nerve. Gradual improvement came, but a lopsided smile still lingers, despite surgery and botox treatments bringing significant progress. Synkinesis—that unpredictable muscle movement—posed a true struggle, but since starting Botox, symptoms have eased. These involuntary, simultaneous movements brought unexpected surprises: muscle pulling, eye twitching, and at times, the face freezing in awkward positions.

Physical therapy followed, bringing the greatest challenge. Imagine a personal trainer pushing limits—that's how demanding these sessions proved. Regaining full strength became the primary mission, starting with relearning to walk. This fueled my anticipation and determination before each appointment. I wanted to be at the gym doing what I loved!

A DVD featuring the last Zumba class before surgery was handed to the physical therapist as motivation—after all, dancing again stood at the heart of recovery. A thoughtful class member and friend brought a tripod to capture that special class on video, not knowing this workout would be the start of making exercise videos. As I handed the physical therapist the DVD, I declared, "This is what I must be doing!"

The therapist gladly accepted the challenge and promised to watch it that evening. Through it all, the mission for healing remained clear to everyone involved.

At my first post-op appointment after brain surgery, stepping into the waiting room was unforgettable. Faces like mine—beautiful, brave, and imperfect—filled the space, each story written in the curve of a smile or an eye that wouldn't quite cooperate. Many were navigating facial paralysis just as I was. An idea to bring us together bubbled up instantly; there ought to be a club.

While Wade and I waited, God sparked an idea in my heart. Why not turn this experience into a way to encourage others? The word "shine" lit up my mind, inspired by Matthew 5:16. *"Let your light shine before others, that they may see your good deeds and glorify your Father in heaven"* (NIV). In that waiting room, God reminded me: keep smiling, keep shining for Him.

My smile didn't have to be perfect; my mission was to point others to Jesus, regardless of my face's symmetry.

That's how the "Shine" T-shirt was born. Since then, sharing these shirts has become a ministry—each one a declaration of courage and hope, especially for those living with facial paralysis. My heart soared the day I gave a shirt to a precious young woman I met on Instagram. She'd always posted workout photos without ever showing her face. After receiving her shirt, she posted a photo—face and all—radiating joy. That moment told me God's message had taken root. The goal isn't just about T-shirts; it's about banishing shame with God's shine.

The journey still brings its challenges, but this is what I know—it's not about how perfect a smile looks, it's about letting Christ's light shine through every struggle, turning sorrow into strength, and shame into radiant, God-given shine.

Years later, social media opened the door to connections I never imagined. Through Facebook and Instagram, I met incredible friends who also live with facial paralysis—including a dear friend born with it with whom I co-founded a private support group. In this safe space, we share our personal journeys, encourage one another, and exchange insights on procedures and treatments that may offer hope. Several members banded together to author a book called *The Hunt for My Smile,* now available on Amazon. If you or someone you love would like a community of encouragement, please reach out to me on Facebook. We welcome new friends with open arms.

Walking through this ongoing trial has taught me to fight for what truly matters, to give my best, and to believe in the possibility of healing. Most of all, finding a supportive community has been a cornerstone in my journey, reminding me that together we can shine brighter and lift each other toward hope.

Reflections

1. Do you have friends who have been through the same difficulties as you? Make a list of those people and send them a text or handwritten note to express your gratitude. You will bless them and in turn be blessed even more!

2. Has God given you an idea to help others? How did that make you feel? Do you feel like there may be more to it than you thought?

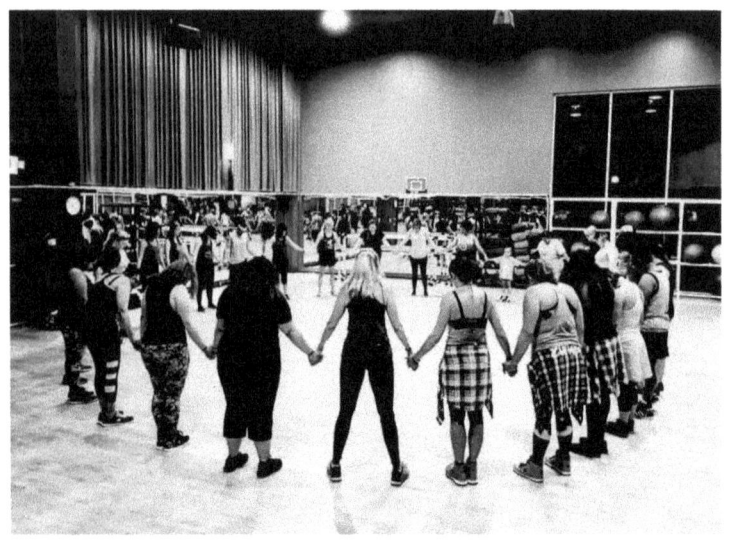

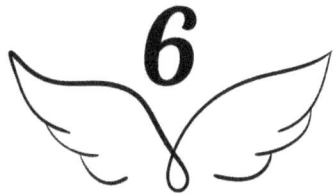

Healing at the Gym

*D*etermination fueled every step of recovery; getting stronger and teaching classes again became a mission. Just six weeks after surgery, the gym doors opened once more. Dizziness persisted, and balance had yet to return, so Wade faithfully drove, and with gentle encouragement, propped me in a spot against the wall, my dumbbells in hand.

When working on a fitness goal, presence in the gym sets the tone. If the goal is healing and fitness, get in the environment where transformation happens. Whether by working out online, hiring a trainer, or joining classes, commitment makes the difference.

Years of teaching at the YMCA fortified an unwavering hope that healing would come, because Jesus is the healer and deserves all the glory. Returning to the gym felt spirit-led; Psalm 37:4 echoes as a promise: God gives us the desires of our hearts. Within eight weeks, teaching weights and spin classes resumed, and four weeks later, the first post-surgery Zumba class arrived as a benefit for a child with a brain injury. Zumba demands choreography, memory, and energy, yet everything clicked—especially during the song "Shackles" by Mandisa. The joy I felt in my heart and spirit radiated out to the whole room; that joy was palpable.

Not everything sparkled, though. On stage, I noticed a small group of women whispered, snickered, and eventually left the dance floor. Their judgment caught me by surprise. My focus shifted, however, to those still dancing, smiling, trying something new, celebrating movement.

Over time, my strength returned. One evening, in the middle of class, my friend Diane called out, "I see more of Angel's teeth!" The once lopsided smile grew wider, evidence that dancing and joy really do help with healing. To this day, my smiles appear brightest after teaching or exercising. Truly, the joy of the Lord provides strength.

A year later, life hummed along, normal as ever. Then came the annual MRI—and devastating news. The tumor had grown back and was larger than before. Dr. Thompson explained that, despite efforts during surgery to seal off the tumor's oxygen, regrowth occurred. Radiation became the next step. Dr. Cmelak in Franklin mapped out a plan: targeted radiation—a specially made mask for precision treatment—in hopes that the tumor, "Tilly," would be evicted.

During each radiation session, the radio played quietly in the background. Pat Benatar's "Hit Me With Your Best Shot" played, and prayers rose that the radiation would strike only the tumor and leave healthy tissue unharmed. After twenty-seven treatments, release came, just in time for a family Cub Scout trip.

But celebration quickly turned to heartbreak. After a day of waterpark fun and a nice hot shower, I began brushing my hair, looking in the hotel mirror. To my horror, hair began to come out in huge clumps. In just a few strokes, the right side of my head was completely bald. The doctor's warnings, now real, brought a wave of emotion. Hair, so often taken for granted, carried a piece of identity. Losing it felt like losing more than the familiar; it became another layer in the struggle to feel beautiful and remain anchored in purpose.

The challenge was far from over. Illness followed: weeks of fever, chills, and sickness drove home the lingering effects of radiation. In bed, support from friends and family—meals, childcare, and a clean house—brought comfort. "Streams in the Desert," a devotional about suffering with Christ, became an inspiration. Suffering now made sense in a new way; God's presence felt deeper than ever, even as black spots marked my face and the threat of tooth loss loomed.

Thirty days later, an MRI delivered more discouragement: tumor growth persisted. Another thirty days, another scan. This time, a friend from church,

Barbara Ann Jeter, organized a prayer watch. Every three hours, loved ones lifted prayers, setting alarms through the night in faithful intercession. The memory still inspires tears—evidence of love, faith, and the real power of prayer. That next MRI? Tumor shrinkage.

Prayer works. God answers. Just like in Mark 2:3-5 where the four friends carried someone to Jesus for healing, sometimes we need friends to carry us, too. Bible studies, small groups, and neighbors stepped in to embody Christ's love. It's never easy to receive help, but sometimes God positions us there on purpose so others can serve and be blessed as well.

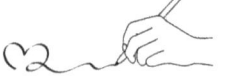 *Reflections*

1) Think about your support system, and how they may have played a key role at crucial times in your life. Take time to thank God for each person He has placed in your life as part of this system.

2) Early on in my healing, I learned I had to disregard negative people and focus on positive support. Have you ever been in

a situation where a handful of "haters" made it difficult for you to focus and achieve your goals? How did you overcome their negativity?

3) Are you in a healing environment? If you want to get better, put yourself where you need to be. Do you need to leave a certain environment?

4) Journal some changes that could help you heal.

Proclaiming health & holiness

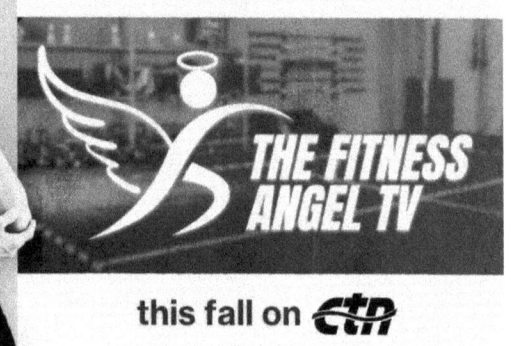

THE FITNESS
ANGEL TV

www.ctntv.org

this fall on

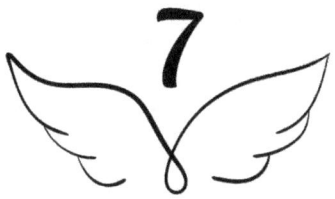

7

Turning Trials into Triumph–Fit to Praise!

*E*merging from those seasons of challenge and healing, a newfound boldness began to develop. Music had always been a foundation in my classes, especially Christian music, but something deeper stirred. No longer content to merely inspire movement, a desire to share Jesus Himself moved to the forefront. Everyone deserved to know my Savior, my Healer; wrapping faith into every beat and every lyric became a natural extension of worship.

When Diane from my spin and Zumba classes asked me to speak at her ladies' Bible study group, a fresh door opened. It was the first time my entire testimony unfolded before an audience, props in hand and praise in my heart. God met me in the sharing—preparing and equipping me for new roles, speaking at women's retreats and events, pouring out His love and power to anyone ready to receive. There, I witnessed what only God could do: hope springing up, passion igniting, and women longing for more of Him in their lives.

Healing wasn't just physical. I also began my quest for true wellness—mind, body, and spirit. Years of teaching fitness didn't mean much if nutrition lagged behind, so I dived into resources about plant-based diets and whole food nutrition. Determined to rewrite our family's habits and give my children the best start, I sought guidance. A chance encounter with a pediatric nurse led to a wellness event, and soon after, a life-giving community at the Christian coffeehouse, Sodium. There, teaching fitness and faith went hand-in-hand. Christian tank tops, T-shirts, and a new motto:—"Fit to Praise"—blossomed. My classes became ministries; women found freedom and joy, and hearts turned to God.

God wasted nothing. Every trial, every class, and every connection became a testimony to His goodness. Invitations to speak and lead "praise parties" grew, stretching from Tennessee to Colorado, Florida, and Pennsylvania—even to Christian TV. Looking back, it's clear. God wove setbacks and victories, laughter and tears, into something that could reach others far beyond what I ever imagined.

A favorite Scripture comes alive as I reflect:

"And we know that in all things God works for the good of those who love him, who have been called according to his purpose."
Romans 8:28, NIV

Every step—through hardship, healing, and hope—proved that with God, nothing is wasted.

The same is true for you; there is purpose in every pain, beauty in redemption, and the power of your story is part of the greater story God longs to tell.

Little did I know the TV show would lead to more open doors in the future!

The retreat weekend in Pennsylvania before the TV appearance taught me to trust God wholeheartedly and to be led by the Holy Spirit when things don't go as planned. When my Pennsylvania retreat host handed me the weekend schedule, my jaw dropped. Right there in her basement apartment, I discovered I was speaking for three sessions instead of one!

Panic bubbled up, so I did the first thing that sprang to mind—called my best friends for emergency backup. Their response? Laughter and love: "You've got this! God will help you fill the time and then some."

Next I called Wade, who couldn't resist a little humor. He teased, "If it were me, I'd be on the next plane back to Nashville! But you? You can talk about Jesus forever." His confidence and that well-timed joke broke the tension and turned worry into excitement.

Armed with my big study Bible (something told me I'd need it!), I sat down, prayed, and set to work organizing three sessions-worth of faith stories, practical wisdom, and encouragement. When the time came to share, splitting my journey across each session turned out to be exactly what the women needed. We laughed, shared, cried, and even ran over on time—God took over and did what He does best! He filled our hearts with hope and courage, reminding us that

His grace can transform even the darkest moments into testimonies of triumph and joy.

After the retreat wrapped up, the limo arrived to take me to the hotel by the TV station. It was my first experience riding in a limo and staying in an upscale hotel all alone! I flopped on the bed with a big smile on my face, soaking it all in and thanking God for all He was doing.

The next morning I was taken to the TV station, a mix of nerves and expectancy in my heart. Sharing my testimony in front of large cameras and a larger audience felt both surreal and humbling. But that day, God made it clear; the story He was writing wasn't just for one group but for women all over the world, anyone ready to hear about His faithfulness. As the interview wrapped up, the host showed me another set. That's where I led an energetic Christian dance fitness class. I was on fire for God and wanted all the viewers to feel the same joyful energy!

The pleasantly-surprised host led me to a long table on another side of the set. The viewers had been calling in and asking for prayer. Hundreds of prayer requests, written on cards, were brought in and dumped on a large table. The gigantic camera zoomed in on me, and the host asked me to pray over all those requests. In that moment, a deep sense of purpose flooded my heart. I felt privileged—what an honor to lift up real people and their needs to the Father right there on live TV. I also felt glad I had seen this done on Christian TV before so I would know what to do.

Putting my hands over the cards, I prayed sincerely, letting God's love and compassion flow. I prayed for healing over the viewers, I prayed for wisdom, finances, families to be restored, freedom from addiction, and deliverance from Satan's schemes and attacks. There in the studio, God's presence felt tangible; those prayers connected hearts across miles, united in hope and belief that God was at work.

This experience became a beautiful reminder that He can use any platform—whether a gym, a retreat, or a TV studio—to touch lives, bring comfort, and spread the message of healing and redemption. Every step, every story shared, builds a bigger picture of God's care; every time I say yes, He multiplies the hope far beyond what I could have imagined. When I surrendered my life to God, I became His vessel.

Say YES and trust the LORD! He can do so much more than we can think or imagine. Never limit God! Matthew 19:26 makes it clear, "*with God all things are possible*" (NIV).

Just as the lights dimmed on my first TV interview and that chapter wrapped up, God surprised me with a fresh opportunity, reminding me that new beginnings often arise on the heels of a remarkable experience. A friend from a Facebook group called "Christians Who Love Zumba" sent me a YouTube link to a song called "Dance Like David." Instantly, inspiration struck—not just from the uplifting music, but from the idea: how amazing would it be to create a Christian fitness DVD? Acting on that spark, I reached out to the song's producer through YouTube, and to my delight, Vincent replied with a wholehearted yes. As we connected, he shared his faith journey, and it became clear that both of us felt called to glorify God through our talents and stories, bringing faith and fitness together for God's kingdom.

The heart behind the DVD was deeply personal. I wanted the proceeds to benefit Best Buddies, a nonprofit supporting kids with disabilities inspired by Scotty, my joyful friend with Down syndrome who never missed a Saturday Zumba class. Around the same time, I was nominated in a fundraising competition for Best Buddies. Their mission is to help children and adults with disabilities feel included, connected, and empowered to reach their full potential. Creating a DVD felt like a meaningful way to contribute. When a friend's husband (who produced kids' TV shows) brought his camera crew to the YMCA, we transformed my vision into a living, breathing project.

Soon after, I created a second DVD—this time focusing on strength training. My neighbor's son, then a college film student, assembled a crew and elevated the project further. Each time someone purchased a DVD, I would pray over the package, trusting that whoever received it was meant to be blessed by the faith-filled music and workout!

Looking back, it's now so clear how these unexpected connections, creative collaborations, and heartfelt intentions became a training ground for my future in television. Every project prepared me for the teamwork, creative vision, and community impact my TV show would require. The experience of turning ideas into reality—and always seeking ways to serve others laid the perfect foundation for what came next in my journey.

God unexpectedly led me into another season of growth and preparation. A friend who was a corporate health coach and took my Zumba class, approached me with encouragement. She believed my passion for wellness and motivating others would translate beautifully to health coaching and invited me to apply for a role with her company.

At that point in life—with a son in high school, a daughter in college, and my health finally restored—my spirit was ready for a new adventure. My faith and fitness ministry brought fulfillment, but I sensed it was time to offer even more to my family, especially after witnessing my husband's years of hard work and selfless provision. The opportunity to become a health coach felt like both a calling and a way to contribute more tangibly.

Embracing this new chapter, I dove into health coaching, quickly discovering that so many of the skills I'd cultivated—listening, teaching, motivating, and cheering others on—translated perfectly to the role. Walking alongside clients as they set goals, overcame obstacles, and celebrated victories brought deep satisfaction and sharpened my ability to connect, communicate, and coach—skills that would become invaluable for television and for growing my own coaching business. The relationships built, lessons learned, and confidence gained in this unexpected detour became the finishing touches to my preparation, ensuring I was fully equipped for the doors God would soon open. This season as a health coach didn't just bridge the gap between ministry and media; it filled me with a new sense of purpose, strengthened my voice, and proved God's faithfulness yet again—always working behind the scenes, preparing me for more than I could ever ask or imagine.

After almost a year in the corporate health coaching position, a deeper truth became undeniable. I was an entrepreneur at heart. The training and skills I gained during that season were invaluable, but I missed the freedom and creative autonomy that had always made me come alive. The wellness company specializing in plant-based nutrition had reached out to me with an opportunity right before the pandemic—I committed to giving it a hundred percent and climbed to the top level, empowered to lead others and share my passion for health in a way that felt authentic and purpose-driven.

I was in a community where health and wellness were valued, and I am grateful God gave me this opportunity. I enjoyed the online community, education, and personal growth, as well as working with my friends who joined me on the quest to share health and wellness with more plant foods!

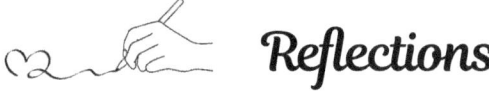 *Reflections*

1) God called me to step out in faith when He gave me a vision. Can you think of a time when you stepped out in faith? If so, how did it feel?

2) There is a season for everything, and God uses everything for His purpose! Reflect on a time when you went through a challenging season, but you could still see God's hand in every step.

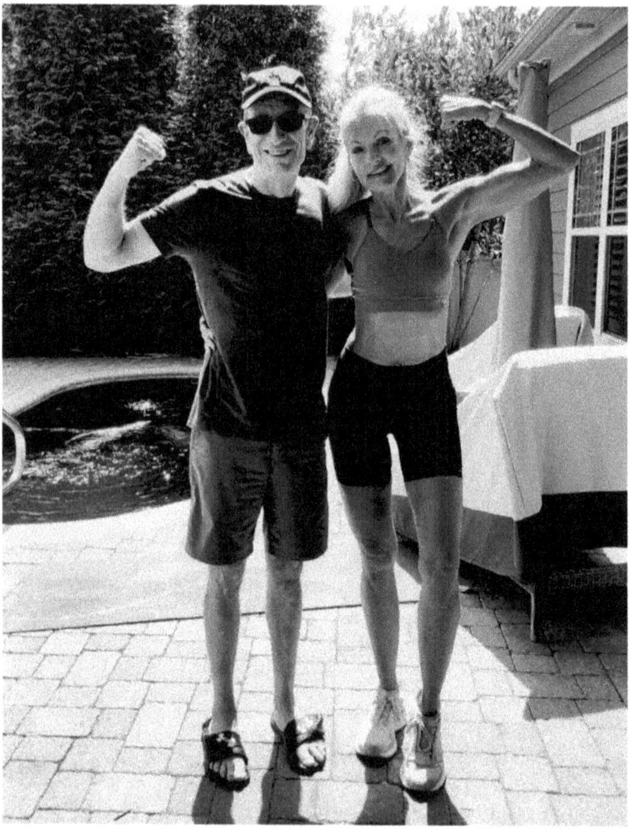

8

A New Season–
Loss to Life and the Gift
of Fresh Beginnings

*D*uring the COVID-19 pandemic, our once-bustling home grew quiet as Wade and I became empty-nesters. Downsizing and moving from the place where we'd built decades of memories was bittersweet, especially after recently losing our two beloved dogs. Still, I wanted Wade to find fulfillment in this new chapter just as I had in the past.

The move was tougher than expected. With soaring home prices and houses selling in a flash, we found ourselves in a new town that felt foreign. I missed our familiar community, church, gym, and routines. On top of that, menopause struck, bringing physical and emotional challenges I'd never faced before. I found myself with no children or pets to care for, no community to pour into, and even my wellness business lacked the energy and excitement it once had. Our adult children were suffering in their own ways. It was as if a dark cloud hung over our family, country, and the world. I felt hopeless, without purpose.

Thankfully, God intervened and met me in my lowest season. Amid the darkness, Lydia returned home, determined to lean on faith and health, and together we started healing. Walks, talks, and a shared focus on God brought us back to life! Our discussions on our daily reading from God's Word, church sermons, fitness, and health goals, pulled us out of the pit and gave us hope for the future. Soon, two new rescue dogs—Jack and Tater Tot—brought laughter back into our home, and our son, Ethan, began flourishing in his new engineering career and returned to making music with his friends.

As Lydia and I reclaimed our health, she introduced me to food logging and calorie tracking, and I combined that with all I'd gained as a health coach and my in-depth research on menopause. Incorporating simple new habits, I surpassed my original goal—reaching my college weight and getting in the best shape of my life—post menopause! Lydia lost eighty pounds, and I lost thirty pounds!

That journey inspired me to create a comprehensive coaching program for women facing similar midlife challenges. My program is rooted in three powerful pillars: nutrition, fitness, and mindset. I teach women how to nourish their bodies with whole food nutrition, how to strength-train for lasting results, and most importantly, how to shift their mindset to break free from old patterns. I provide a supportive community where we set goals, celebrate victories, and encourage each other every step of the way. The women who follow my coaching program lose inches, pounds, and body fat, as well as gain muscle, energy, confidence, and a renewed sense of purpose—improving not only their bodies but their whole lives.

As our circle grew, so did my calling to give back. That's when I launched my own charity to fund my TV show, *The Fitness Angel TV*. We share faith, fitness, and health all over the world to help women improve every area of their lives—body, mind, and spirit! The Lord has blessed us so we can bless others.

The doors God has opened—a thriving coaching program, a dynamic TV show launching soon, and now a mission-driven charity—are proof that every chapter, trial, and triumph served as preparation for this ministry. I am living evidence that, no matter your age or starting point, you can reclaim your health, hope, and happiness.

> *"Dear friend, I pray that you may enjoy good health and that all may go well with you, even as your soul is getting along well."*
> 3 John 1:2, NIV

If you feel stirred by this message, I invite you to join me. Please reach out on social media, visit my website, and connect with our community. Allow me to encourage you on your journey with Jesus! If you feel led, please partner with me on this mission to share faith, fitness, and health with the world through Christian television! Together, we can make an even bigger impact through uplifting women, building strong bodies and spirits, and showing the world the strength, joy, and peace that come from walking with God.

Remember, it's never too late for a fresh start, and you're not alone. Let's embrace new beginnings together, inspire change, and carry the message of hope to every woman, one transformed life at a time. The best is yet to come!

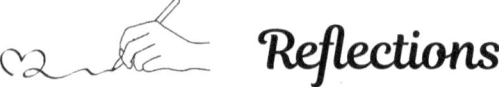 **Reflections**

1) Throughout my life challenges, God has demonstrated His presence with overwhelming love. Think of a time when you felt God's presence during a difficult period. How did you know He was with you?

2) Take time to journal about this experience. And remember, He will never leave or forsake you (Hebrews 13:5).

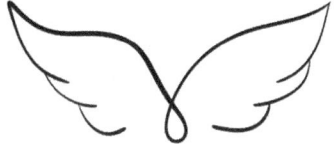

About the Author

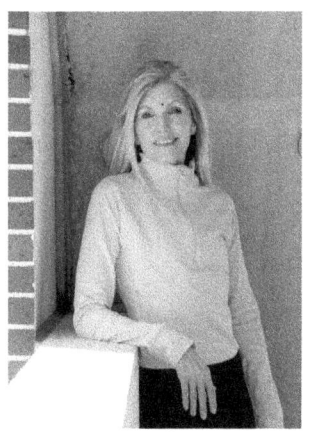

Angel Faulk has been married to her husband, Wade, for 32 years. Together they are the proud parents of Ethan, Lydia, and their son-in-law Josh. With a degree in education and experience teaching elementary school, Angel ultimately followed her true passion as a faith-filled fitness and health expert.

Known as The Fitness Angel, she has created Christian fitness DVDs and recently launched her new program, *The Fitness Angel TV*. Angel also coaches women online, helping them navigate the challenges of menopause and step into the best shape of their lives—body, mind, and spirit.

She loves speaking at women's events, sharing her testimony, and leading joyful "praise party" fitness classes that combine faith, fun, and fitness.

You can connect with Angel at thefitnessangel.net or find her on Facebook, Instagram, YouTube, and TikTok.

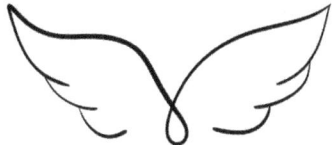

Acknowledgments

First and foremost, I give thanks to my Lord and Savior, Jesus Christ, for guiding me, giving me strength, and blessing this journey. All glory belongs to Him.

To my husband, Wade—thank you for your unwavering love, patience, and encouragement through every season of life. To Ethan and Lydia, and my son-in-law Josh—you bring so much joy to my heart, and I am grateful for your support and belief in me.

To my MAMMA, who is smiling down from heaven—thank you for being my greatest cheerleader. Your love and encouragement continue to inspire me every day.

To my coaching clients—you inspire me every day. Walking alongside you on your health and fitness journeys has been one of the greatest blessings of my life.

To the doctors, mentors, and friends who have guided, supported, and prayed for me along the way—your wisdom, care, and intercessions mean more than words can express.

To everyone who has supported *The Fitness Angel TV* and helped us share fitness, faith, and health on Christian television, I am deeply grateful.

To all the pastors, churches, and women's groups where I have had the privilege of speaking, leading fitness classes, and sharing my testimony —you remind me daily that this mission is bigger than myself.

Finally, to everyone who has cheered me on, encouraged me, and believed in this vision— thank you from the bottom of my heart. And for those who follow my journey, stay tuned … my next book will share our path to justice, a story of faith, perseverance, and hope.